Trout Cookbook

Tasty & Simple Trout Recipes

BY

Stephanie Sharp

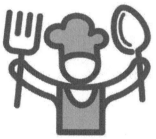

Copyright © 2019 by Stephanie Sharp

License Notes

Copyright 2019 by Stephanie Sharp All rights reserved.

No part of this Book may be transmitted or reproduced into any format for any means without the proper permission of the Author. This includes electronic or mechanical methods, photocopying or printing.

The Reader assumes all risk when following any of the guidelines or ideas written as they are purely suggestion and for informational purposes. The Author has taken every precaution to ensure accuracy of the work but bears no responsibility if damages occur due to a misinterpretation of suggestions.

wwwwwwwwwwwwwwwwwwwwwwww

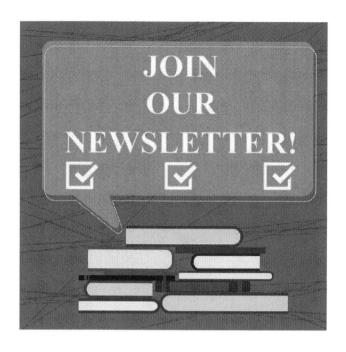

My deepest thanks for buying my book! Now that you have made this investment in time and money, you are now eligible for free e-books on a weekly basis! Once you subscribe by filling in the box below with your email address, you will start to receive free and discounted book offers for unique and informative books. There is nothing more to do! A reminder email will be sent to you a few days before the promotion expires so you will never have to worry about missing out on this amazing deal. Enter your email address below to get started. Thanks again for your purchase!

Just scan QR-code to get started!

Table of Contents

Introduction 8

   Trout, Avocado and Grapefruit Salad 9

   Spice Crusted Trout 12

   Trout and Barley Salad 14

   Grilled Trout 17

   Fusilli Trout 19

   Trout Skewers 22

   Trout Quiche 24

   Grilled Trout Peaches 27

   Smoked Trout Risotto 30

   Trout Tartar 33

   Trout Cannelloni 36

   Trout and Ricotta Pie 39

   Thai Style Trout Noodles 42

Broiled Trout Parmesan 45

Trout Noodle Soup 47

Curried Trout 50

Trout Soup with Wild Rice 52

Trout and Broccoli Stir Fry 55

Whole Meal Pasta with Smoked Trout 57

Trout and Mozzarella Stacks 59

Trout Stew 62

Baked Whole Trout 65

Stuffed Baked Trout 69

Trout Curry 72

Poached Trout 75

Trout in Yogurt Marinade 77

Trout Ricotta Roll 79

Trout and Pea Stew 82

Smoked Trout Spanish Omelet and Potatoes 84

Cajun Trout Burgers 87

Conclusion 90

About the Author 91

Author's Afterthoughts 92

Introduction

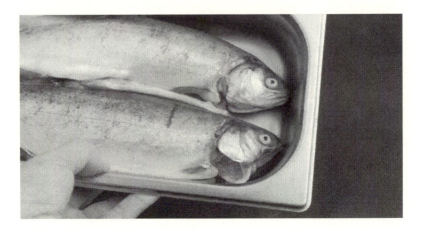

For an interesting and delicious meal that requires a short time or effort, cook up some juicy trout! Trout is by far a crowd favorite when it comes to freshwater fish. You can grill it, fry it or bake it! There are various ways to cook trout. You can customize your meal to suit your nutritional needs and tastes. Trout can be a beautiful addition to a two-course meal for family or dinner guests, or it can be a simple treat after a long day at work. These 30 delectable and nutritious recipes were put together just for you. Enjoy!

Trout, Avocado and Grapefruit Salad

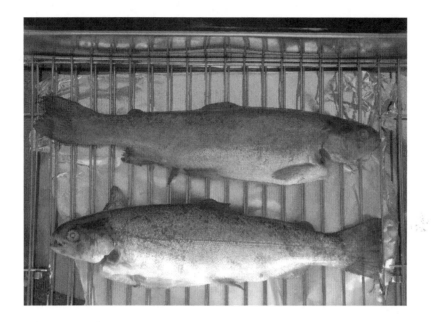

Not only is this recipe nutritious but with its tangy, fresh and rich ingredients, it is a sophisticated alternative. The crunch of the walnuts enhances the softness of the trout fillet.

Serves: 4

Time: 30 mins.

Ingredients:

- 16 oz. of boneless fresh Trout Fillet
- 1 sliced ripe Avocado
- 1 Grapefruit
- 2 bunches of Rocket without their stems
- ¼ cup of toasted chopped Walnuts
- 3 tbsp. of Olive Oil
- 2 tbsp. of Lemon Juice
- ½ tsp of Salt
- ½ tsp of Pepper

Directions:

1. Begin by peeling the grapefruit. Separate into segments and remove skin.

2. Place the grapefruit in a bowl. Add the rocket and avocado.

3. Whisk the lemon juice, 2 tbsp. of oil and ¼ tsp of salt together. Add the pepper.

4. Season the trout with remaining salt and pepper.

5. Heat 1 tbsp. of olive oil in a frying pan over medium heat. Add the trout and cook for 4 minutes on each side or until cooked through.

6. Remove from the pan and break up into pieces.

7. To serve, place the salad into bowls. Lay the trout on the salad and top with walnuts. Drizzle with the lemon juice mixture. Enjoy!

Spice Crusted Trout

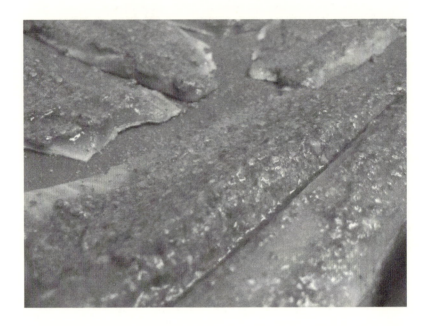

It's a simple recipe, but it's also a very special and tasty one!

Serves: 4

Time: 25 mins.

Ingredients:

- 1 teaspoon fennel seeds
- 1 teaspoon mustard seeds
- 4 medium trout steaks
- ¼ teaspoon black peppercorns
- A pinch of sea salt
- Black pepper to the taste
- 4 tablespoons sesame seeds
- 3 tablespoons coconut oil

Directions:

1. In your grinder, mix peppercorns with fennel and mustard seeds and grind well.

2. Add sesame seeds, a pinch of sea salt, and pepper to the taste and grind again well.

3. Spread this mix on a plate, add trout steaks and toss to coat.

4. Heat up a pan with the oil over medium high heat, add trout steaks and cook for 3 minutes on each side.

5. Divide between plates and serve with a side salad.

6. Enjoy!

Trout and Barley Salad

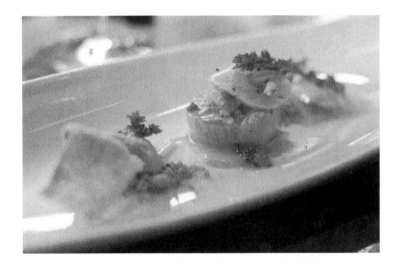

Barley accompanies trout perfectly in this salad. The dressing is zesty and fresh. Served with vegetables, it makes a complete and healthy meal.

Serves: 4

Time: 40 mins.

Ingredients:

- 21 oz. of skinless and boneless Trout Fillet
- ½ cup of Pearl Barley
- 2 stalks of thinly sliced celery
- ½ finely sliced Cucumber
- ½ cup of Plain Yogurt
- ¾ cup of chopped Fresh Parsley
- 2 tbsp. plus ¼ cup of chopped Fresh Dill
- 4 tbsp. of Lemon Juice
- 1 tsp of Lemon Zest
- 3 tbsp. of Olive Oil
- 2 tsp of Dijon Mustard
- Salt, to taste
- Pepper, to taste

Directions:

1. Start by preheating the oven to 425 degrees F and lining a baking tray with foil.

2. Place the barley and 1.5 cups of water in a pot. Bring to the boil and add some salt.

3. Reduce heat to low, cover and cook for 25 minutes or until barley is tender. Drain any left-over water and spread the barley on a baking sheet.

4. Whisk 2 tbsp. of lemon juice, mustard and 1 tbsp. of oil in a bowl.

5. Add the parsley, 4 tbsp. of dill and lemon zest.

6. Place the trout on the lined baking tray and spread the herb mixture over it.

7. Put the trout in the oven for 12 minutes or until the trout has cooked through.

8. Meanwhile, whisk the yogurt with the remaining lemon juice, olive oil and dill. Add salt and pepper to taste.

9. Add the celery, cucumber and barley to the bowl and mix.

10. To serve, place the barley mixture on plates and top with flaked pieces of cooked trout. Enjoy!

Grilled Trout

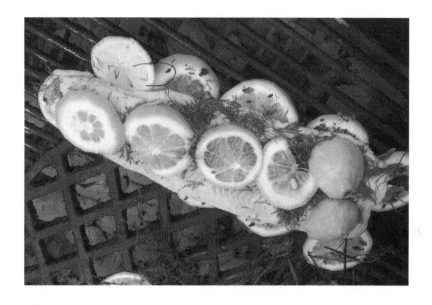

Get your servings of Omegas in with this tasty fish dish.

Serves: 2

Time: 35 minutes

Ingredients:

- 2 trout fillets
- ½ teaspoon garlic paste
- 3 tablespoons lemon juice
- 1 teaspoon salt
- ½ teaspoon black pepper
- ½ teaspoon oregano
- 1 teaspoon fish sauce
- ¼ teaspoon turmeric powder
- 2 tablespoons olive oil

Directions:

1. Sprinkle turmeric powder on fish and rub all over. Leave it for 10-15 minutes then wash out fish well.

2. Take a bowl add vinegar, lemon juice, pepper, salt, fish sauce and oregano, toss to combine.

3. Spread this mixture on fish fillets and rub on it with hands.

4. Preheat grill and spray with oil. Place fish fillets on grill and let to brown well.

5. Flip the side and make sure both sides are cooked well.

6. Serve and enjoy.

Fusilli Trout

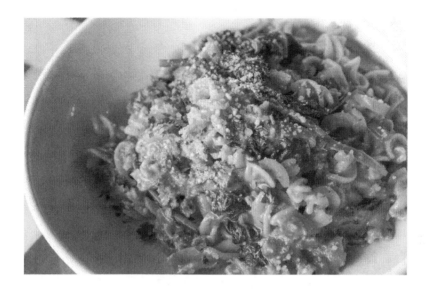

This lovely pasta is tasty and simple, yet at the same time extremely satisfying. It is easy and quick to make, as well as being delicate and interesting.

Serves: 4

Time: 20 mins.

Ingredients:

- 1 lb. of fusilli (spirals)
- 7 oz. of diced Fresh Trout
- 1/3 cup of Cooking Cream
- 1 ¼ cup of Tomato Puree
- 2 oz. of Diced Black Olives
- ½ tsp of Oregano
- 1 tsp of Minced Dill
- 2 cloves of minced Garlic
- 3 tbsp. of Olive Oil
- Salt, to taste
- Pepper, to taste

Directions:

1. Start by heating a large pot of water for the pasta.

2. Heat the olive oil in a large pan on low setting. Add the garlic and cook until fragrant.

3. Add the olives and trout to the garlic and cook for 3 minutes.

4. In another pan, heat the tomato puree and the cream and bring to the boil.

5. Add the herbs and the salt and pepper to taste. Set aside.

6. When the water for the pasta has boiled, add salt followed by the pasta. Cook until al dente.

7. Mix the pasta with the creamy puree and the trout mixture and serve.

8. Enjoy!

Trout Skewers

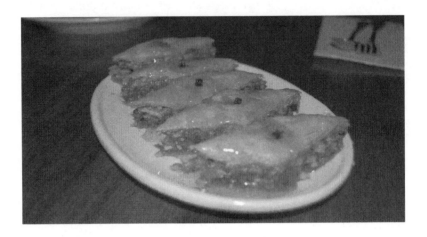

These are so fresh and easy to make!

Serves: 4

Time: 25 mins.

Ingredients:

- 1-pound wild trout, skinless, boneless and cubed
- 2 Meyer lemons, sliced
- ¼ cup balsamic vinegar
- ¼ cup orange juice
- 1/3 cup Paleo orange marmalade
- A pinch of pink salt
- Black pepper to the taste

Directions:

1. Heat up a small pot with the vinegar over medium heat, add marmalade and orange juice, stir, bring to a simmer for 1 minute and take off heat.

2. Skewer trout cubes and lemon slices, season with a pinch of salt and black pepper, brush them with half of the vinegar mix, place on preheated grill over medium heat, cook for 4 minutes on each side.

3. Brush skewers with the rest of the vinegar mix, grill for 1 minute more, divide between plates and serve.

4. Enjoy!

Trout Quiche

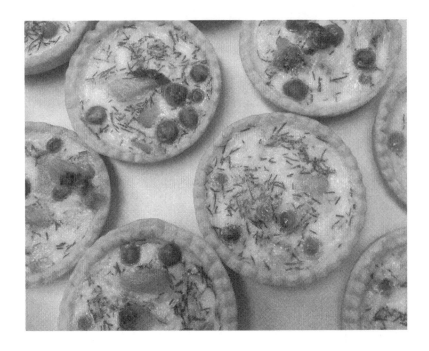

Beautiful and colorful, this quiche will not disappoint. It is simple to make and can be part of a larger meal.

Serves: 4

Time: 1 hr. 15 mins.

Ingredients:

- 2 cups of cooked Trout
- 3 Eggs
- 1 cup of Flour
- 1 cup of grated Parmesan
- ½ cup of Milk
- 1 cup of Sour Cream
- 6 tbsp. of Olive Oil
- ¼ cup of Mayonnaise
- 1 tbsp. of chopped Fresh Chives
- ¼ tsp of Paprika
- ¼ tsp of Hot Sauce
- Salt, to taste
- Pepper, to taste

Directions:

1. Begin by preheating the oven to 350 degrees F and line a round pie or quiche pan.

2. Place the flour in a bowl. Add half the parmesan, olive oil, salt and paprika and combine well.

3. Press the mixture onto the bottom and sides of the pan and bake for 10 minutes.

4. Reduce oven to 330 degrees.

5. Meanwhile, beat the eggs in a bowl. Add milk, sour cream, mayonnaise, chives, hot sauce and salt and pepper to taste.

6. Add the flaked pieces of Trout and the remaining parmesan and pour into the baked crust.

7. Bake in the oven for 50 minutes or until completely cooked.

8. Remove from the oven and cool.

9. To serve, cut into slices and accompany with an herb salad.

10. Enjoy!

Grilled Trout Peaches

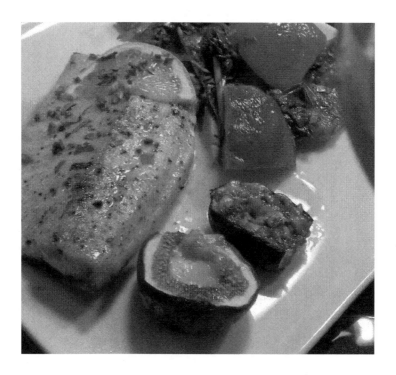

Try this combination as soon as possible! It's really amazing and easy to make!

Serves: 4

Time: 25 mins.

Ingredients:

- 2 red onions, cut into wedges
- 3 peaches, cut in wedges
- 4 trout steaks
- 1 teaspoon thyme, chopped
- 1 tablespoon ginger, grated
- A pinch of sea salt
- Black pepper to the taste
- 1 tablespoon white wine vinegar
- 3 tablespoons extra virgin olive oil

Directions:

1. In a bowl, mix wine with ginger, vinegar, thyme, a pinch of sea salt, pepper and olive oil and whisk very well.

2. In a bowl, mix peaches with onion, salt and pepper and toss to coat.

3. Heat up your kitchen grill over medium high heat, add trout steaks after you've seasoned them with pepper to the taste, grill for 6 minutes on each side and divide between plates.

4. Add peaches and onions to grill, cook for 4 minutes on each side and transfer next to trout on plates.

5. Drizzle the vinaigrette you've made all over trout, onions, and peaches and serve right away. Enjoy!

Smoked Trout Risotto

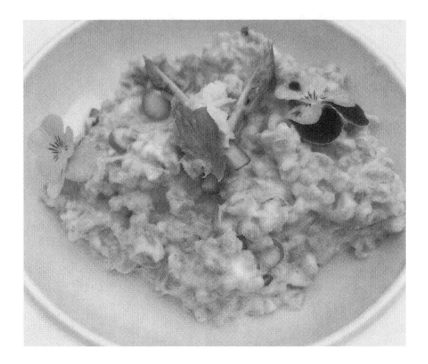

Who can resist a risotto? This recipe combining the creaminess of Arborio rice with the smokiness of the smoked trout is a great meal to share with friends.

Serves: 4

Time: 30 mins.

Ingredients:

- 9 oz. of Arborio Rice
- 3.5 oz. of finely diced Smoked Trout
- ½ finely diced Red Onion
- 1.5 oz. of Butter
- ½ glass of Dry White Wine
- ¾ cup of Tomato Puree
- 1 pinch of Hot Paprika
- grated Zest of 1 Lemon
- Salt, to taste

Directions:

1. Start by cooking the rice according to the package's instructions.

2. Meanwhile, melt the butter in a large pan and add the onions. Cook until the onions brown.

3. Add the trout and then the wine to the onions. Allow the wine to evaporate.

4. Add the tomato puree, paprika and salt to the pan. Cook on low heat for 5 minutes.

5. When the rice is cooked, drain it and add it to the pan. Stir thoroughly for 5 minutes.

6. Serve the risotto sprinkled with the lemon zest. Enjoy!

Trout Tartar

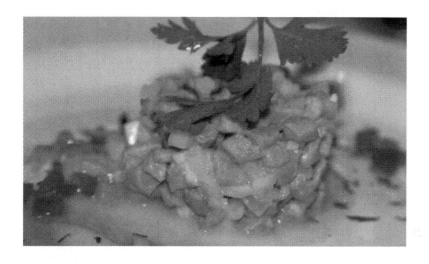

This is a good idea for a party appetizer! It's really good!

Serves: 4

Time: 15 mins.

Ingredients:

- 7 ounces smoked trout, minced
- 14 ounces trout fillet, cut into very small cubes
- 3 tablespoons red onion, minced
- 2 tablespoons pickled cucumber, minced
- Zest and juice from 1 lemon
- 1 garlic clove, finely minced
- 2 tablespoons basil, minced
- 2 teaspoons oregano, dried
- Black pepper to the taste
- 2 tablespoons mint leaves, minced
- 2 tablespoons Dijon mustard
- 5 tablespoons extra virgin olive oil
- Lime wedges for serving

Directions:

1. In a bowl, mix onion with cucumber, garlic, lemon zest and juice, basil, mint, oregano, mustard, oil and pepper and stir well.

2. Add smoked and fresh trout and stir well again.

3. Divide tartar between plates and serve with lime wedges on the side.

4. Enjoy!

Trout Cannelloni

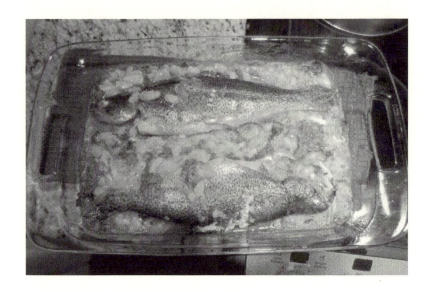

This beautiful pasta dish combines the delicacy of ricotta and béchamel sauce with the smoked trout. It is a high protein dish. Followed by a salad, this dish makes a complete meal.

Serves: 4

Time: 40 mins.

Ingredients:

- 10 sheets of approximately 4 x 2 in Fresh Lasagna Dough
- 5 oz. of diced Smoked Trout
- 7 oz. of Ricotta
- ¾ cup of Béchamel Sauce
- 1 Egg White
- ½ bunch of minced Parsley
- ¼ a cup of Bread Crumbs
- ½ cup of grated Parmesan
- 1 oz. of sliced Butter
- Salt, to taste
- Pepper, to taste

Directions:

1. Begin by preheating the oven to 400 degrees F and line an oven proof tray with wax paper.

2. Carefully lay out the pasta sheets onto a flat floured working surface.

3. Place the trout in a bowl. Add ricotta, a handful of parmesan and salt and pepper to taste.

4. Stir the trout and ricotta mixture until it becomes smooth. Add the egg white.

5. To prepare the cannelloni, spoon the trout mixture into the middle of the lasagna sheet and roll it. Place it on the tray and repeat until you have used up all the sheets. Make sure the cannelloni are lying close to each other.

6. Cover the cannelloni with béchamel sauce.

7. Sprinkle the remaining parmesan, the bread crumbs and butter.

8. Cook in the oven for 30 minutes or until a crusty surface has formed.

9. Remove from the oven and sprinkle with parsley to serve.

10. Enjoy!

Trout and Ricotta Pie

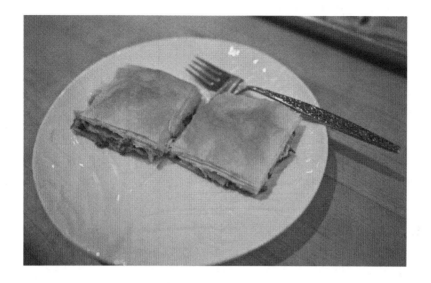

This gorgeous pie is refined in taste. The subtlety of ricotta blends beautifully with the smoked Trout. Served with warm vegetables, it makes a complete and healthy meal.

Serves: 4

Time: 1 hr.

Ingredients:

- 7 oz. of Smoked Trout
- 1 sheet of Short Crust Pastry
- 3 Eggs
- 7 oz. of Ricotta
- 1.5 oz. of Feta
- ½ cup of grated Parmesan
- 1 bunch of chopped Fresh Parsley
- Salt, to taste

Directions:

1. Begin by preheating the oven to 350 degrees F and greasing a pie dish.

2. Combine ricotta, half the parmesan and feta in a bowl. Mix to make a smooth consistency.

3. Add the parmesan and mix well.

4. Beat the eggs and add to the cheese mixture.

5. Dice the Trout and add to the bowl.

6. Place the pastry onto the pie dish. Poke holes with a knife.

7. Pour the mix into the pie dish. Sprinkle the top with remaining parmesan and bake for 40 minutes or until the crust has started to turn golden.

8. Remove from the oven and cool.

9. Serve with a fresh tomato salad. Enjoy!

Thai Style Trout Noodles

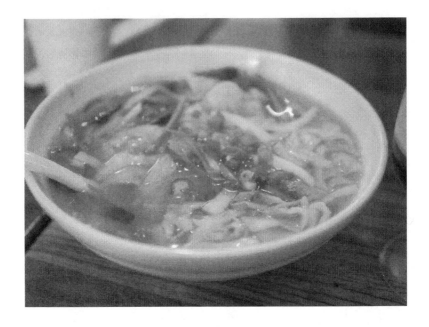

This Thai inspired recipe is brimming with flavor. The sauce accompanies the trout wonderfully.

Serves: 4

Time: 40 mins.

Ingredients:

- 14 oz. of skinless and boneless Trout Fillet cut into strips
- 7 oz. of Rice Noodles
- 1 medium sized Sweet Potato
- 3 tsp of Thai Red Curry Paste
- 1 tsp of Vegetable Oil
- ¾ cup of Vegetable Stock
- ½ cup of Skimmed Milk
- 2 chopped Spring Onions
- Small bunch of chopped Coriander

Directions:

1. Start by boiling water in a large pot.

2. Cook the noodles according to the instructions on the package. Rinse them and drain them. Set them aside.

3. Heat oil in a frying pan. Once hot, add your curry paste then cook for one minute.

4. Add the spring onions, milk, stock and sweet potato and bring to the boil. Simmer the heat and cook until the sweet potato is soft.

5. Add the trout and cook for another 3 minutes.

6. Turn off the heat and stir through half of the coriander.

7. To serve, place the noodles in bowls.

8. Top with trout and sauce and sprinkle with the remaining coriander. Enjoy!

Broiled Trout Parmesan

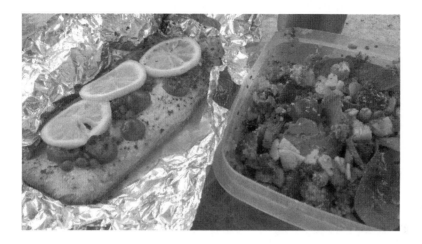

This Trout Parmesan is a play on the traditional chicken parmesan. It is quick and delicious.

Time: 15 m

Serves: 8

Ingredients:

- Trout (4 lbs., boneless, cut into thin pieces)
- Salt (2 tsp., to taste)
- Garlic Powder (1 tsp.)
- Onion Powder (½ tsp.)
- Paprika (¼ tsp.)
- Pepper (1 tsp., to taste)
- Parmesan Cheese (1 cup, grated)

Directions:

1. Preheat your broiler to 400 degrees F.

2. Season your trout to taste, then set to broil until your fish has been fully cooked through (about 10 minutes).

3. Top with parmesan and return to broiler until your parmesan has melted, spread, and lightly browned. Enjoy!

Trout Noodle Soup

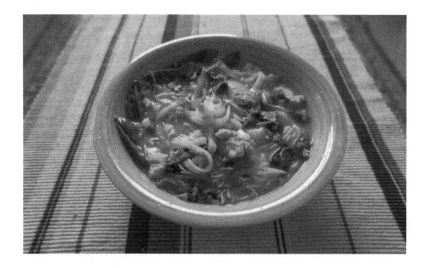

The coconut milk lends such richness to the broth while the lemongrass and lime juice add a beautiful freshness. All this enhances the flavor of the trout.

Serves: 4

Time: 40 mins.

Ingredients:

- 2 cloves of chopped Garlic
- 1 chopped large Onion
- 2 peeled and chopped Lemongrass Stalks
- 1 tbsp. of Vegetable Oil
- 4 FL oz. of Coconut Milk
- 7 FL oz. of Fish Stock
- 8 oz. of diced Skinless and Boneless Trout Fillets
- 4/5 oz. of Rice Noodles, cooked
- 1 tsp of Turmeric
- 1 tsp of hot Chili Powder
- 7 oz. of Fresh Bean Sprouts
- 1 quartered Lime
- 1 small bunch of Coriander
- Salt, to taste
- Pepper, to taste

Directions:

1. Start by bringing a large pot of water to the boil.

2. Make a paste by blending the lemongrass with the onion, turmeric and chili powder.

3. Heat the oil on a large frying pan.

4. Fry the paste for 4 minutes until fragrant.

5. Stir in the coconut milk and then the fish stock.

6. Bring to the boil and then simmer for 15 minutes with a lid.

7. Add the trout and continue to cook with a lid for 5 more minutes or until the trout is cooked.

8. Add the bean sprouts and cook for 1 more minute.

9. To serve, place the noodles in bowls and top with the trout soup. Garnish with the lime and coriander. Enjoy!

Curried Trout

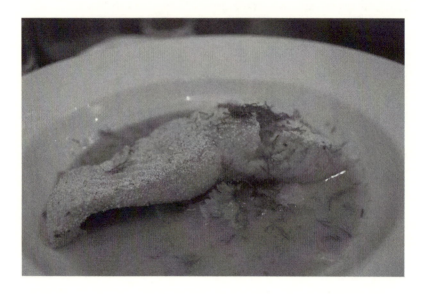

If you have never tried curried fish, then this may be the recipe for you.

Serves: 4

Time: 8 hours 10 minutes

Ingredients:

- 1 teaspoon ground coriander seeds
- 2 tablespoons yellow curry paste
- 4 garlic cloves, minced
- 1 lb. trout, rinsed and dried then cubed
- ½ lb. green beans, cut into ½-inch pieces
- 1 cup finely chopped brown onion
- 4 small carrots, chopped
- 2 medium potatoes, cut into ½-inch slices
- ½ teaspoon cayenne pepper
- 1 ½ cup fish stock
- 1 cup coconut milk
- 1 tsp. Fresh ground salt and pepper

Directions:

1. Add your curry in a saucepan with oil over medium heat and cook until fragrant (about a minute).

2. Add in your fish and allow to lightly brown in curry for about 2 minutes per side.

3. Combine all your remaining ingredients.

4. Cover and cook on medium for 20 minutes.

5. Season to taste, serve, and enjoy.

Trout Soup with Wild Rice

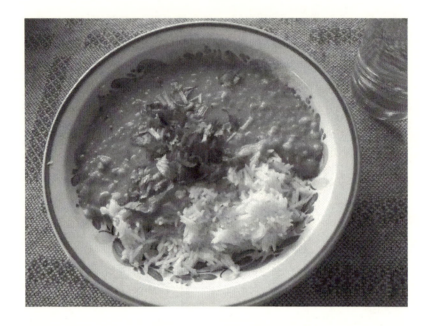

While fresh trout can be used for this recipe, canned trout adds a very different touch to this soup. It is a perfect choice for those winter nights when it is too cold outside.

Serves: 4

Time: 40 mins.

Ingredients:

- 3 oz. of Canned Trout
- 2 cups of Wild Rice
- 3 cups of Vegetable Broth
- 2 tbsp. of Vegetable Oil
- ½ cup of Cooking Cream
- 1 diced medium sized Onion
- 1 cup of Diced Celery
- 1 cup of sliced Mushrooms
- 7 FL oz. of Vegetable Stock
- ½ cup of Cream
- 2 tbsp. of Flour
- Salt, to taste

Directions:

1. Begin by boiling water in a large pot. Add salt when boiling.

2. Add the wild rice and cook until tender. Drain.

3. Meanwhile, heat oil in another large pot.

4. Add the onion and the celery and cook for 5 minutes.

5. Add the mushroom and the stock and simmer for 15 minutes.

6. Add the trout and salt to taste and cook for 5 minutes.

7. Meanwhile, combine the flour and cream.

8. Add the cream and flour mixture to the pot.

9. Then add the cooked rice

10. Turn off heat when the flour mixture is cooked through. Enjoy!

Trout and Broccoli Stir Fry

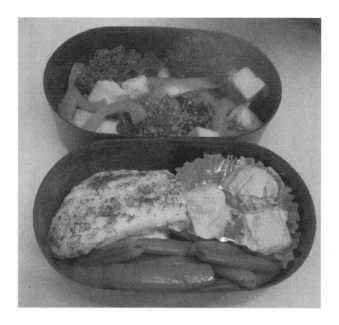

Astonishingly simple, this stir fry makes a perfect healthy and complete meal. The broccoli complements the trout beautifully. It can be served over rice or noodles.

Serves: 4

Times: 15 mins.

Ingredients:

- 14 oz. Fresh Trout Fillet
- 7 oz. of Broccoli
- 4 diced Spring Onions
- 2 crushed cloves of Garlic
- 5 tbsp. of Water
- 2 tbsp. of Thai Fish Sauce
- 4 tbsp. of Soy Sauce

Directions:

1. Begin by heating a wok.

2. Add the water garlic, spring onions and broccoli. Stir fry for 4 minutes.

3. Meanwhile cut the trout into strips.

4. Add to the wok with the fish sauce and soy sauce.

5. Stir gently and cook for 3 minutes or until the trout is cooked.

6. Serve over brown rice. Enjoy!

Whole Meal Pasta with Smoked Trout

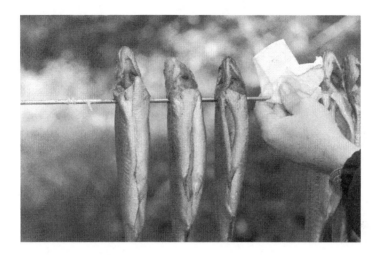

This recipe is quick and easy to make. It is best served at room temperature so the mozzarella does not melt in the heat of the pasta.

Serves: 6

Time: 40 mins.

Ingredients:

- Smoked Trout, 4.5 oz.
- Buffalo Mozzarella, 9 oz.
- 1 lb. of whole meal Short Pasta
- 1 tbsp. of Olive Oil
- 1 bunch of chopped Parsley
- 1 bunch of Basil
- Salt, to taste
- Pepper, to taste

Directions:

1. Start by boiling water in a large pot.

2. Add salt when the water boils, cook the pasta until al dente and drain. Set aside.

3. Meanwhile, cut the mozzarella and the trout into small cubes.

4. Mix the oil, pepper, basil and parsley together. When the pasta is at room temperature, pour the oil and herb mixture into it. Mix well.

5. Add the trout and the mozzarella and toss again.

6. Serve the pasta at room temperature. Enjoy!

Trout and Mozzarella Stacks

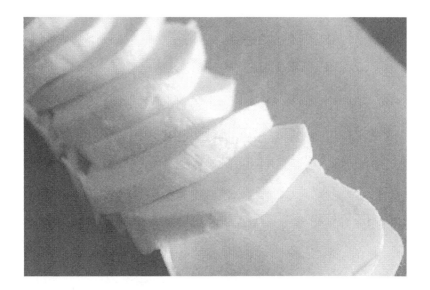

This recipe is aesthetically beautiful and at the same time deliciously wonderful. The melted cheese will please any child who may not be a fan of eating fish.

Serves: 4

Time: 40 mins.

Ingredients:

- 14 oz. of Smoked Trout
- 14 oz. of Fresh Mozzarella
- 5 medium sized Potatoes
- 4 tbsp. of Olive Oil
- 1 tbsp. of Oregano
- Salt, to taste
- Pepper, to taste

Directions:

1. Begin by preheating the oven to 400 degrees F and line a baking tray with wax paper.

2. Peel the potatoes and slice them very thinly.

3. Put them in a bowl and season them with 2 tbsp. of olive oil, salt, pepper and oregano.

4. Place them on the baking tray and cook in the oven for 20 minutes until they have become crisp.

5. Remove from the oven.

6. Assemble the stacks by laying the potatoes on a plate, followed by a topping of trout and one of mozzarella. Continue layering in this way until you have reached the height you prefer.

7. Drizzle with olive oil.

8. Just before serving, heat the stacks in the oven to melt the cheese. Enjoy!

Trout Stew

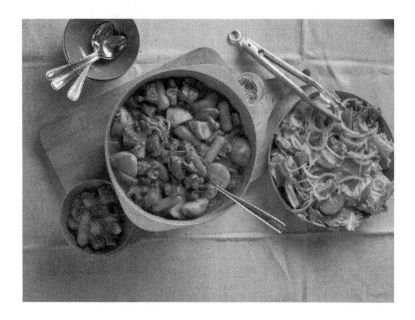

This trout stew is a great idea for the winter evenings. It can be served with rice or barley or other grain of choice.

Serves: 4

Time: 1 hr. 10 mins.

Ingredients:

- 1 lb. of fresh skinless and boneless chunks of fresh Trout
- 12 oz. of cooked Chick Peas
- 4 diced Tomatoes
- 1 small diced Onion
- 2 cups of canned Roma Tomatoes
- 1.5 cups of pitted Olives of choice
- 4 tbsp. of Olive Oil
- pinch of Paprika
- 1 bunch of Coriander
- Salt, to taste
- Pepper, to taste

Directions:

1. Start by heating 2 tbsp. of olive oil in a large frying pan.

2. Add the onions and cook until they are soft.

3. Add tomatoes and cook for 10 minutes.

4. Add chickpeas, olives and coriander, cover and simmer for another 5 minutes.

5. Brush the trout with the remaining olive oil, salt, pepper and paprika.

6. Lay the trout over the sauce and cook for 40 minutes with the lid on.

7. Serve hot with a side of rice. Enjoy!

Baked Whole Trout

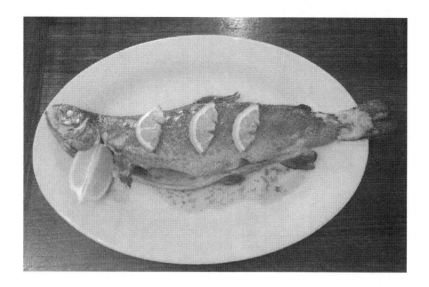

This trout recipe is elevated by the infusion of herbs. The trout can be served with potato salad or roasted potatoes.

Serves: 10

Time: 1 hr. 15 mins.

Ingredients:

- 1 Whole Trout (4 lb.)
- 5 FL oz. of Vegetable Broth
- ½ a finely diced Onion
- 3 thinly sliced Lemons
- 4 tbsp. of Olive Oil
- 1 tbsp. of Wholegrain Mustard
- 2 tsp of Honey
- 1 bunch of Rosemary
- 5 Bay Leaves
- 1 bunch of Fresh Dill
- Salt, to taste

Directions:

1. Begin by preheating the oven to 400 degrees F and grease a baking tray with 1 tbsp. of olive oil.

2. Scatter the rosemary, bay leaves and lemon slices along the base of the pan.

3. Use a sharp knife to make 1.5-inch cuts on both sides of the fish.

4. Season the trout with salt.

5. Place the fish on the bed of herbs and lemon. Drizzle with 2 tbsp. of olive oil and bake in the oven for 35 minutes or until the fish is cooked through.

6. Meanwhile, to make the mustard sauce, heat the remaining tbsp. of olive oil in a small pan. Add the onion and cook on low heat for 8 minutes.

7. Add the stock lemon and salt to taste and simmer for 5 minutes.

8. Remove the trout from the oven.

9. Add the mustard, honey and dill to the onion mixture in the pan.

10. To serve, remove the skin of the trout and slice into fillets. Drizzle fillets with the warm mustard sauce and accompany with potato salad. Enjoy!

Stuffed Baked Trout

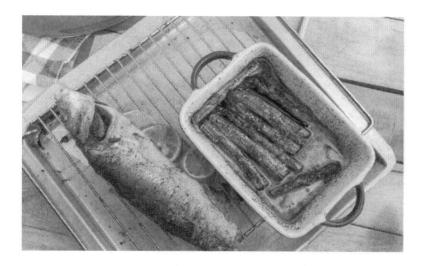

The leek stuffing gives the trout a sweetness that is irresistible. This recipe makes a healthy filling meal.

Serves: 4

Time: 50 mins.

Ingredients:

- 1 25 oz. piece of Fresh Trout Fillet
- 2 medium sized Leeks
- Juice and zest of 1 Lemon
- 2 tbsp. of Olive Oil
- 1 tbsp. of Butter
- 1 tbsp. of Soy Sauce
- 1 minced clove of Garlic
- Salt, to taste
- Pepper, to taste

Directions:

1. Begin by preheating the oven to 350 degrees F and lining a baking tray with wax paper.

2. Chop the leeks into thin rounds.

3. Heat1 tbsp. of olive oil and the butter in a pan. Add the leeks and cook on low heat for 20 minutes.

4. Add salt to taste and stir regularly.

5. Remove from heat and allow to cool.

6. Meanwhile, using a sharp knife, cut into the middle of the trout fillet to create an area to stuff.

7. Place trout onto the baking tray.

8. Combine the lemon juice, lemon zest olive oil, soy sauce and garlic in a bowl and pour over the trout.

9. Fill the trout fillet with the leek mixture.

10. Bake in the oven for 15 minutes or until the trout is cooked through.

11. Serve the trout with baked potatoes. Enjoy!

Trout Curry

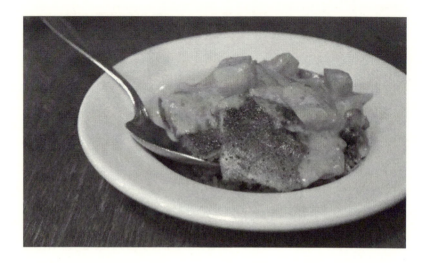

The spices in this recipe give the trout a depth and unexpected surge of flavor. It is beautiful with rice but can also be served with flatbread.

Serves: 6

Time: 45 mins.

Ingredients:

- 24 oz. of chunks of Trout Steak
- 1 in of chopped fresh Ginger
- 1 Onion
- 3 cloves of minced Garlic
- 3 chopped Green Chili
- 2 chopped Tomatoes
- ½ cup of strained Greek Yogurt
- ½ cup of fresh Fenugreek Leaves
- 2 tbsp. of chopped Coriander
- 3 tbsp. of Vegetable Oil
- 1 tsp of Turmeric
- 1 tsp of Cumin Seeds
- 4 green Cardamom Pods
- 2 Cloves
- 4 cm Cinnamon Stick
- 1 tsp of Salt
- 1 tsp of Sugar

Directions:

1. Begin by rubbing the trout with salt and turmeric.

2. Combine tomatoes, onion, ginger and garlic in a bowl.

3. Heat the oil in a pan on medium heat. Add the cumin seeds, cardamom pods and cloves. Break the cinnamon stick into pieces and add to the pan. Cook for 30 seconds. Add the tomato mixture to the pan. Cook for 15 minutes.

4. Carefully add the trout and ½ cup of water to the pan and simmer for 10 minutes.

5. Meanwhile, beat the yogurt and sugar together. Stir the fenugreek leaves and the coriander. Add to the trout curry and simmer for 5 minutes without boiling.

6. Serve over rice. Enjoy!

Poached Trout

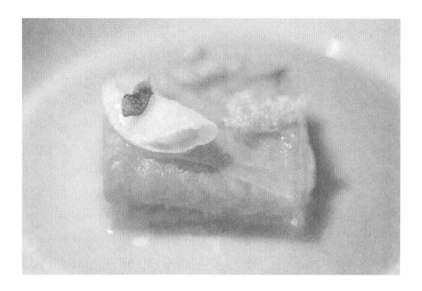

Poaching trout is a wonderful alternative. It goes well with mashed potatoes but also with a healthy salad.

Serves: 4

Time: 7 mins.

Ingredients:

- 25 oz. of Trout Fillets
- 1 juiced Lemon
- ½ cup of Water
- ½ cup Dry White Wine
- 2 tbsp. of Butter
- 1 clove of minced Garlic
- 2 tbsp. of chopped Fresh Parsley
- Salt, 1 tsp.

Directions:

1. Begin by melting butter in a large frying pan.

2. Add the garlic and cook for 1 minute.

3. Add the trout to the pan. Season with salt and pepper and brown the fish on both sides for 1 minute.

4. Add the water and white wine to the pan and cover. Cook for 5 minutes.

5. Pour the lemon juice over the fillets.

6. Serve with mashed potatoes.

Trout in Yogurt Marinade

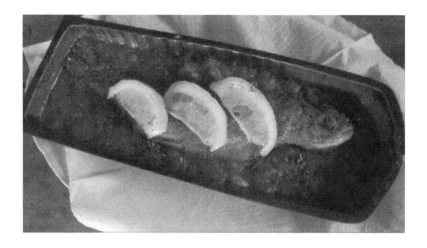

This recipe is delicious and has a beautiful crusty layer which combines very well with mashed potatoes for a healthy and filling meal.

Serves: 4

Time: 55 mins.

Ingredients:

- 2 lb. of fresh Trout Cutlets
- 2 cups of Plain Yogurt
- 6 tbsp. of Soy Sauce
- Juice of 1 Lemon
- 4 tbsp. of Worchester Sauce
- 2 tbsp. of Vegetable Oil.

Directions:

1. Begin by mixing together the yogurt, Worchester sauce and lemon juice.

2. Place the trout cutlets onto a tray and cover with the yogurt marinade.

3. Place the trout in the refrigerator for 30 minutes.

4. Heat the oil in a large nonstick frying pan.

5. Place the trout in the pan and increase heat to high. Cook for 1 minute and then flip it on its other side.

6. Continue to cook until the trout has formed a crust.

7. Serve with mashed potatoes. Enjoy!

Trout Ricotta Roll

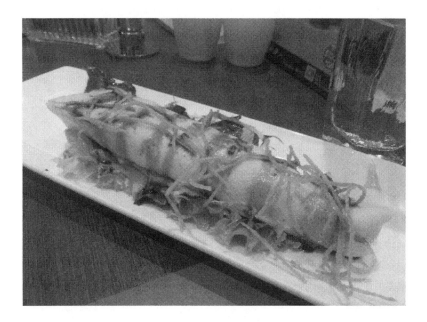

This Argentinian recipe is great for the summer. It is both light and filling with all the nutrition of trout. It can be served with a warm or cold salad.

Serves: 4

Time: 25 mins.

Ingredients:

- 7 oz. of cooked skinless and boneless Trout Fillet
- 3 Eggs
- 3 tbsp. of Flour
- 3 tbsp. of Sugar
- 5 oz. of Cream Cheese
- Ricotta, 3.5 oz.

Directions:

1. Start by preheating the oven to 350 degrees F and lining a baking tray lined with wax paper.

2. Beat the eggs with the sugar until they become pale and thick.

3. Sift the flour into the eggs and stir carefully trying not to lose the volume created.

4. Gently spread the egg mixture onto the tray and bake for 10 minutes.

5. Remove the dough from the oven and lay it flat onto some wax paper. Cover it with a wet tea towel and roll it together with the wax paper. Set aside to cool.

6. Meanwhile, mix the ricotta and cream cheese together until smooth.

7. When the dough has cooled, lay it flat again.

8. Spread the cheese mixture onto it.

9. Arrange the trout slices over the cheese and roll again.

10. Let it rest and then cut into slices.

11. To serve, place some slices onto a plate and accompany with a green salad. Enjoy!

Trout and Pea Stew

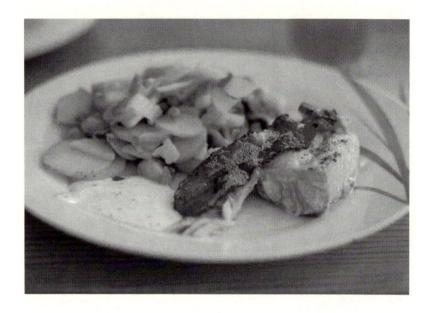

Trout and peas accompany each other wonderfully in this hearty and easy to prepare stew. Great for the winter, it is a comforting and complete meal.

Serves: 4

Time: 35 mins.

Ingredients:

- 2 lb. of skinless and boneless Trout Fillet
- 2 cups of Vegetable Broth
- 21 oz. of Sweet Peas
- 1 diced Onion
- 2 tbsp. of Olive Oil
- Salt, to taste
- Pepper, to taste

Directions:

1. Start by heating the broth in a pot.

2. Add the peas, salt and pepper and cook for 10 minutes or until peas are cooked through.

3. Meanwhile, cut the trout into 1-inch chunks.

4. Add the trout to the pot of peas and cook for another 10 minutes.

5. Serve the stew with a side of rice. Enjoy!

Smoked Trout Spanish Omelet and Potatoes

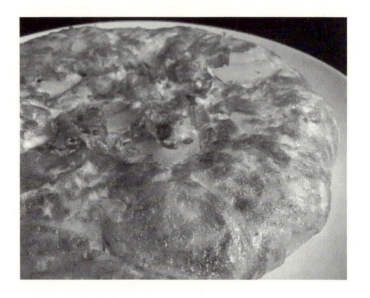

This beautiful egg and trout recipe are a hearty meal packed with plenty of flavor.

Serves: 4

Time: 1 hr. 30 mins.

Ingredients:

- 7 oz. of sliced Smoked Trout
- 5 unpeeled diced medium sized Potatoes
- 6 Eggs
- 1 thinly sliced Onion
- 1 head of Roasted Garlic
- 4 tbsp. of chopped Fresh Parsley
- 4 tbsp. of Olive Oil
- 1 tbsp. of Butter
- Salt, to taste
- Pepper, to taste

Directions:

1. Start by preheating the oven to 400 degrees F and line a baking tray.

2. Place the potatoes on the tray. Drizzle with 2 tbsp. of olive oil and salt and pepper.

3. Bake potatoes in the oven for 25 minutes until they have become brown and soft.

4. Meanwhile, heat 1 tbsp. of olive oil and the butter in a pan. Add the onion, salt and pepper and cook over medium heat for 30 minutes until they have become caramelized.

5. Remove from the pan and set aside.

6. Beat the eggs with salt and pepper.

7. Heat the same pan used for the onions. Add 1 tbsp. of olive oil, roasted garlic and the roasted potatoes and stir.

8. Add the eggs, cooked onions, smoked trout and parsley.

9. Cook on medium heat with a lid for 20 minutes.

10. Slide the omelet onto a plate and flip it back into the pan to cook on the other side. Enjoy!

Cajun Trout Burgers

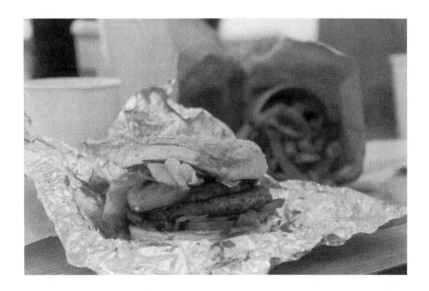

This burger is seasoned with Cajun spices and is made of trout meat. These burgers can be eaten in a bun or served with a side salad or potatoes.

Serves: 5

Time: 45 mins.

Ingredients:

- 1 lb. of shredded skinless and boneless Trout Fillets
- 2 Eggs
- ½ cup of Breadcrumbs
- 1 bunch of chopped Fresh Parsley
- 2 tsp of minced Garlic
- Half diced Onion
- ½ tsp of Thyme
- 1 tbsp. of Cajun Seasoning
- ¼ tsp of Hot Sauce
- 2 tbsp. of Olive Oil
- Salt, to taste
- Pepper, to taste

Directions:

1. Begin by preheating the oven to 400 degrees F and grease a baking tray with the olive oil.

2. Combine the thyme and parsley in a bowl. Add Cajun seasoning, breadcrumbs, hot sauce, onion, garlic, and salt and pepper to taste.

3. Mix thoroughly.

4. Add the trout to the bowl.

5. Beat the eggs lightly and transfer to the bowl.

6. Mix until very well combined.

7. Using your hands, use the trout mixture to make burger shapes.

8. Place the burgers on the baking tray and bake for 15 minutes.

9. Serve in a bun with salad or accompanied by a baked potato. Enjoy!

Conclusion

Congrats on cooking your way through all 30 delicious Trout recipes that can all be enjoyed at any Trout lover. The next step from here would be to continue practicing. With every single Trout recipe, you create you will see magic being created as you go through this book.

After you have accomplished that, come on back over and find another amazing journey to partake in from cuisines across the globe in another one of our books. We hope to see you again soon.

Happy cooking!

About the Author

Born in New Germantown, Pennsylvania, Stephanie Sharp received a Masters degree from Penn State in English Literature. Driven by her passion to create culinary masterpieces, she applied and was accepted to The International Culinary School of the Art Institute where she excelled in French cuisine. She has married her cooking skills with an aptitude for business by opening her own small cooking school where she teaches students of all ages.

Stephanie's talents extend to being an author as well and she has written over 400 e-books on the art of cooking and baking that include her most popular recipes.

Sharp has been fortunate enough to raise a family near her hometown in Pennsylvania where she, her husband and children live in a beautiful rustic house on an extensive piece of land. Her other passion is taking care of the furry members of her family which include 3 cats, 2 dogs and a potbelly pig named Wilbur.

Watch for more amazing books by Stephanie Sharp coming out in the next few months.

Author's Afterthoughts

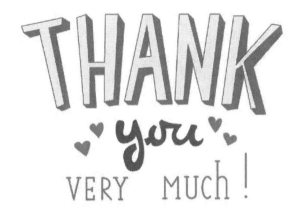

I am truly grateful to you for taking the time to read my book. I cherish all of my readers! Thanks ever so much to each of my cherished readers for investing the time to read this book!

With so many options available to you, your choice to buy my book is an honour, so my heartfelt thanks at reading it from beginning to end!

I value your feedback, so please take a moment to submit an honest and open review on Amazon so I can get valuable insight into my readers' opinions and others can benefit from your experience.

Thank you for taking the time to review!

Stephanie Sharp

Made in the USA
Columbia, SC
05 January 2023